The Bible Cure ®

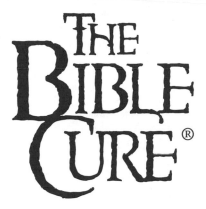

Recipes for Overcoming Candida

Don Colbert, M.D.

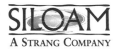

SILOAM

A Strang Company

The Bible Cure Recipes for Overcoming Candida
by Don Colbert, M.D.
Published by Siloam
A Strang Company
600 Rinehart Road
Lake Mary, Florida 32746
www.siloam.com

Unless otherwise noted, all Scripture quotations are from the Holy Bible, New Living Translation, copyright © 1996. Used by permission of Tyndale House Publishers, Inc., Wheaton, IL 60189. All rights reserved.

Scripture quotations marked KJV are from the King James Version of the Bible.

Library of Congress Catalog Card Number:
2003112758

A BIBLE CURE PRAYER
FOR YOU

Lord, I thank You that You desire to restore me to health: spirit, soul and body! Please teach me the things I need to change in my diet and nutritional habits to overcome the overgrowth of candida in my body, and give me strength to apply these principles in my life. In Jesus' name, amen.

As you read and choose to apply and trust God's promises, it will help you to use the powerful Bible Cure prayers I have included to line up your thoughts and feelings with God's plan of divine health for you, a plan that includes living victoriously. In this Bible Cure book, you will discover insights into better health and nutrition in the following chapters:

It is my prayer that these recipes and nutritional tips will help restore wholeness to your life—spirit, soul and body. And may this book also deepen your fellowship with God and strengthen your ability to worship and serve Him.

—DON COLBERT, M.D.

Candida, one type of yeast found within the human intestines, is quite normal and is compatible with a lifetime of excellent health. Its growth is generally held in check by the presence of "good" bacteria also present in the intestines. However, under the influence of various medications, dietary choices and stress, the delicate balance between the good bacteria and candida can become disrupted. Then the once harmless levels of yeast grow out of control and may begin to invade and colonize throughout the body.

This Bible Cure book is filled with nutritional facts, delicious recipes and cooking tips to help you overcome candida. But even more importantly, it will encourage you to stand strong against temptation by the power of God's Word and begin to apply godly principles to your eating habits. In this book, you will

uncover God's divine plan of health
for body, soul and spirit
through modern medicine, good nutrition
and the medicinal power
of Scripture and prayer.

You will also discover life-changing scriptures throughout this book that will strengthen and encourage you.

will help cure these conditions. And in this Bible Cure book, you will discover healthy, nutritious and delicious recipes to help you develop these good nutritional habits. First, I will introduce the basic facts regarding candida to help you make healthy changes in your eating habits.

What Is Candida?

Candida, or the yeast syndrome, is simply an overgrowth of yeast that usually lives in the intestinal tract. But in women it can also manifest in painful infections in the vagina. When yeast overgrows in the GI tract, it can cause a number of distressing symptoms, including heartburn, indigestion, abdominal bloating, cramps, constipation or diarrhea, nausea or gas.

Are you experiencing these symptoms? If so, you may be exhibiting signs of an overgrowth of candida. I suggest that you also read *The Bible Cure Book for Candida and Yeast Infections*. It contains further descriptions of this problem as well as dietary and supplement information that will help you restore balance in your intestinal tract and health throughout your body.

Everyone has various kinds of yeast living on his or her skin and in the intestinal tract.

Restoring Your Health With Nutrition

G od is in the business of restoring His people to health! He promises this in His Word: "'I will give you back your health and heal your wounds,' says the Lord" (Jer. 30:17). His desire is to renew and restore you—body, soul, mind and spirit. The Bible says, "Dear friend, I am praying that all is well with you and that your body is as healthy as I know your soul is" (3 John 2).

Many individuals have healthy souls, but they are living their lives here on earth in sick or weakened bodies. Perhaps you have been weakened or made ill by the effects of candida (yeast) running rampant in your body. If so, take heart! God has provided a way out for you! The most powerful way to combat the effects of yeast imbalances in your body is through the practice of sound, healthy nutritional habits.

In *The Bible Cure for Candida and Yeast Infections*, I explain the nutritional habits that

International Standard Book Number:
0-88419-940-1

04 05 06 07 08 — 987654321
Printed in the United States of America

Chapter 1

Be an Overcomer!

If you have been held captive by the weakening effects of candida overgrowth in your body, it is important for you to realize that *this problem can be overcome!* God is on your side, ready to help. If you turn to Him, He will empower you with the strength you need to be an overcomer in this area of your life.

The Bible tells us that "he gives power to those who are tired and worn out; he offers strength to the weak. Even youths will become exhausted, and young men will give up. But those who wait on the LORD will find new strength. They will fly high on wings like eagles. They will run and not grow weary. They will walk and not faint" (Isa. 40:29–31).

> *I am the LORD who heals you.*
> —EXODUS 15:26

If you are ready and willing to make a change in your life, this Bible Cure book is for you. Rely on God's strength to help you implement the nutritional changes you need to make in your diet—and to follow through with those changes.

First, let's consider briefly the causes and symptoms of this problem—as well as the role that nutrition can play in alleviating it.

Causes and Symptoms

The overgrowth of candida is prevented by "good" bacteria, which are usually present in our colon. However, antibiotics, certain environmental factors, as well as bad nutritional habits, can deplete the amount of good bacteria that are actively working on our behalf. When this occurs, candida begins to grow out of control in the intestinal tract, producing mycotoxins, which are toxins produced by yeast, and potentially causing many serious problems. This yeast overgrowth syndrome is known as *candidiasis.*

Diverse causes

Factors that trigger candidiasis include using antibiotics, birth control pills and corticosteroids prescribed for treatment of disease. Another trigger is eating sugar and highly processed carbohydrates.

Yeast multiplies rapidly in the body by feeding on sugar. The average American consumes 150 pounds of sugar per year. In many cases, that is more than a person's own body weight! When you decide to indulge in desserts such as cakes, pies, cookies, brownies and the like, you are literally inviting the candida in your body to a feast!

Distressing symptoms

Yeast overgrowth is able to produce seventy-nine known toxins. One of the most toxic substances produced by yeast is acetaldehyde. When this substance enters into the liver, it is converted into alcohol. Acetaldehyde contributes to a raft of harmful symptoms, including fatigue, mental cloudiness, disorientation, confusion, irritability, headaches, anxiety and depression.

Not only does yeast overgrowth produce these distressing symptoms, but it also depletes minerals, it increases free radical formation, and it disrupts enzymes the body needs to produce energy.

If the yeast overgrowth continues unchecked, it

> *You must serve only the LORD your God. If you do, I will bless you with food and water, and I will keep you healthy.*
> —EXODUS 23:25–26

can further weaken our immune system, and its mycotoxins may then affect any organ or tissue in the body. As soon as a particular organ in your body is affected, symptoms flair. For instance, as candida or its toxic waste products affect the nervous system, you may begin to experience fatigue, memory loss, insomnia, depression, mood swings, sleepiness, attention-deficit disorder, hyperactivity, or autistic tendencies.

Many diseases and illnesses are usually yeast related, including those listed below:

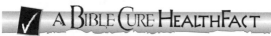

A BIBLE CURE HEALTHFACT

Yeast-Related Diseases and Illnesses

- Chronic fatigue syndrome
- Severe allergies
- Multiple chemical sensitivities
- Endometriosis
- Infertility
- Decreased sex drive
- Eczema
- Rheumatoid arthritis
- Multiple sclerosis
- Recurrent ear infections
- Bronchitis
- Sinusitis
- Attention-deficit hyperactivity disorder
- Food allergies
- Premenstrual syndrome
- Interstitial cystitis
- Sexual dysfunction
- Psoriasis
- Asthma
- Lupus
- Autism
- Most autoimmune disorders
- Fibromyalgia

HEALTHFACT HEALTHFACT HEALTHFACT HEALTHFACT HEALTHFACT HEALTHFACT HEALTHFACT

From the diseases and illnesses listed, you can see that when yeast grows out of control it

4

can weaken the body, wreaking havoc wherever it goes. And the toxins produced by candida can make you feel absolutely miserable.

If you suspect you may be suffering from yeast overgrowth, take the self-test on page 25 to see how you stack up.

The Role of Nutrition

When I discuss the possibility of candida overgrowth with my patients, I usually ask them one very important question: "What foods do you crave?" Most patients with a candida problem have one answer in common: "I crave sugar!"

If you are a person who can't resist cakes, pies, cookies, colas, chocolate, breads, ice cream, alcohol or other processed foods that are high in sugar and carbohydrates, it is time to take control of your eating habits! You are literally feeding the problem. Even some foods that are considered to be healthy, like fruits and fruit juices, can contribute to an overgrowth of yeast in the body.

> *I have heard your prayer and seen your tears. I will heal you.*
> —2 KINGS 20:5

Fortunately, there is a way to eat healthy foods that are high in nutritional content, which will decrease the growth of candida—and they are delicious as well! Keep reading to discover the specially-formulated recipes and nutritional tips designed specifically to reduce candida and put you back on track to a balanced lifestyle and a strong, healthy body.

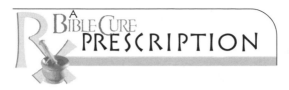

A BIBLE CURE PRESCRIPTION

Are there any foods that you crave? If so, what are they?

_____

_____

_____

_____

Are you willing to make necessary changes in your diet to combat candida overgrowth in your body? If so, pray the following prayer:

Heavenly Father, Your Word says that You will restore my body to health and give me a long, satisfied life. I stand on Your promises today as I begin to confront this problem of candida overgrowth in my body. Thank You for Your wisdom that will show me the specific steps I need to take to walk in health. In Jesus' name I pray. Amen.

Chapter 2

Laying the Ground Rules

Overcoming candida will require you to stay on the candida diet for a period of time. Yet the world we live in constantly barrages us with advertisements for "fast foods," sugar-filled, and highly processed foods. But while discipline must play a key role in maintaining this diet, the good news is that your meals do not have to be boring and dull!

The Bible says, "The joy of the LORD is your strength" (Neh. 8:10); it also tells us to "go ahead.

> O LORD my God,
> I cried out to
> you for help, and
> you restored my
> health.
> —PSALM 30:2

Eat your food and drink your wine with a happy heart, for God approves of this!" (Eccles. 9:7). How can anyone eat their food with a happy heart if their meal is boring, bland or monotonous—if they are following a diet out of drudgery? This book will provide you with simple, delicious recipes that will make it a joy to follow the candida diet.

To begin, we need to establish the following guidelines for a few weeks to ensure your success. If this list of *nos* seems overwhelming to you, let me remind you of the delicious recipes that are waiting for you to try in the next chapters. For now, commit to the following:

1. No sugar of any kind may be consumed on this diet. That includes white sugar, brown sugar, honey, molasses, syrup, sucrose, lactose, maltose, fructose or corn syrup.

2. No artificial sweeteners are allowed, including Sweet'n Low, NutraSweet or Equal. However, Stevia and Splenda are acceptable.

3. No fruit juice is allowed. After the candida is brought under control, a small amount of grapefruit juice may be permitted.

4. No fruit of any kind may be consumed during the first three weeks of the diet. After the third week, some low-sugar fruits may gradually be introduced, such as apples, pears,

kiwis, blueberries, blackberries, raspberries, strawberries, grapefruit, lemons and limes.

5. No lactose is allowed; therefore, no milk, cheese, cottage cheese, ice cream or sour cream is permitted. A small amount of organic butter and yogurt or kefir may be used, as long as it contains no lactose, sugar or fruit.

6. No gluten grains may be eaten. These include wheat, rye, white or pumpernickel breads, as well as pastries, pasta, crackers, etc. Oat products usually contain less gluten and may be eaten by those with less severe candida overgrowth. Grains that are acceptable include brown rice bread or crackers; millet bread; spelt bread, crackers or pasta; and brown rice.

7. No foods containing yeast of any kind are permitted—including bakery products or commercially prepared food products.

8. No alcoholic beverages of any kind may be consumed.

9. No dry roasted nuts are allowed. However, nuts in the shell—other than peanuts, pistachios or cashews—are acceptable, because the shell keeps these nuts from molding.

10. No vinegar or vinegar-containing foods are allowed. (The possible exception would be raw unfiltered apple cider vinegar only for those with mild cases of candida.)

11. No soy sauce, tamari or natural root beer is allowed.

12. No vitamin or mineral supplements containing yeast may be taken.

13. No pickled foods or smoked, dried or cured meats, including bacon, may be eaten. This includes processed lunchmeats, sausage, hot dogs, salami, bologna, etc.

14. No deep-fried foods of any kind are allowed.

15. No mushrooms may be eaten.

16. No caffeinated beverages may be consumed, including coffee, teas and sodas. Instead, choose herbal teas, such as dandelion root tea, pau d'arco, fruit teas or mint tea, but be sure they do not contain citric acid.

17. No corn of any kind may be eaten, including corn on the cob, corn chips, popcorn, corn meal, etc.

18. No refined oils may be used in cooking, including sunflower oil, safflower oil or corn oil. Instead, use cold-pressed oils such as extra-virgin olive oil.

19. Avoid potatoes and sweet potatoes since these are rapidly converted to sugars within the body.

Although these ground rules may seem intimidating at first, if you persevere with these dietary changes, the results in your health and overall energy levels will be dramatic. After about three months of avoiding these foods, many candida patients find that they can gradually re-introduce some of them into their diet, rotating them every three to four days. But some foods should always be avoided for those with a candida problem, including foods that are high in sugar such as sugary desserts, ice cream and alcoholic beverages.

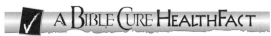

A BIBLE CURE HEALTHFACT

On the nutritional labels of food products, most sugars are the substances that end with the letters "o-s-e."

HEALTHFACT HEALTHFACT HEALTHFACT HEALTHFACT HEALTHFACT HEALTHFACT HEALTHFACT

Strengthening the Immune System

As your immune system grows weaker, the candida in your body has the opportunity to grow stronger. As you begin to follow the candida diet to restore your body to health, it is important to not forget these crucial steps to strengthen your immune system.

- Be sure to get eight to ten hours of sleep each night.
- Take a Sabbath day of rest each week.
- Decrease your stress.
- Take steps to simplify your life.
- Practice having a merry heart!

Supplements Can Help

In addition to getting sufficient rest and reducing your stress levels, it may be helpful to take nutritional supplements to modulate your immune system. Moducare and Natur-Leaf are plant sterols and sterolins, which are helpful for this condition. I recommend taking either Moducare or Natur-Leaf. Moducare is found at most health food stores; the recommended dosage is two capsules in the morning and one in the evening on an empty stomach. Natur-Leaf must be ordered. (See Appendix B for ordering information.) The recommended dosage is one capsule twice a day on an empty stomach or one hour before meals.

> *The Lord nurses them when they are sick and eases their pain and discomfort.*
> —Psalm 41:3

Author's note: For more information on any of these supplements or testing procedures mentioned in this section, refer to Appendix B at the back of this book.

Total Leaky Gut

In addition to supplements that bring balance to the immune system, it can also be helpful to take other nutritional supplements while on the candida diet. To heal damage done to the GI tract, I recommend taking Total Leaky Gut at a dose of one tablet, three times a day, thirty minutes before meals.

Beneficial bacteria

To overcome candida, it is critically important to restore beneficial bacteria to the GI tract. To do this, I recommend multiple forms of beneficial bacterial, including Divine Health Probiotic at a dose of two tablets twice a day on an empty stomach. Three Lac is another excellent probiotic; I recommend one packet twice a day before meals. Finally, Probiotic Pearls, one tablet twice daily, is also important.

> *Lord, your discipline is good, for it leads to life and health. You have restored my health and have allowed me to live!*
> —Isaiah 38:16

Antifungal agents

In addition, an antifungal agent should be taken to reduce the yeast levels in the intestinal tract. For patients with a mild candida problem, I recommend Divine Health Candida Formula, in a dosage of one tablet three times a day.

Some patients may need something stronger,

such as Nystatin, which must be prescribed by a physician.

Other patients are so infested with yeast that they need an even more potent medication such as Diflucan, which must be closely monitored by a doctor.

Biotin

To keep candida in its noninvasive form, most candida patients need to take a supplement of biotin, at a dose of 1,000-microgram capsule three times a day. This nutrient is usually deficient in patients with candidiasis. Biotin may be found in most health food stores.

Help for allergies

Most candida patients have numerous food allergies or sensitivities, and an excellent way to desensitize them is with NAET, a noninvasive, drug-free, natural solution to treat allergies of all types. Their Web site is www.naet.com

You can also determine your food allergies with a blood test such as the ALCAT test. (See Appendix B.)

There may be times when avoiding sugar is impossible. A birthday party, holiday seasons or other celebrations may make it very difficult to pass up foods that you would not ordinarily eat. On those occasions, remember to exercise self-control and take an extra biotin supplement and a natural antifungal agent, such as Divine Health Candida Formula, to counteract the sugars in your system.

More Factors to Consider

Most candida patients can restore health simply by following the candida diet and taking the supplements listed above. However, if after six months your symptoms have still not improved, you should consider the possibility of other contributing factors to your condition. Some of these factors may include the following:

1. *A hormone imbalance.* There may be adrenal, thyroid or sex hormone imbalance present. Many patients with candida suffer from subclinical hypothyroidism and should take a

natural thyroid supplement. Most candida patients also have low adrenal function and require an adrenal supplement such as DSF, one tablet two times a day. (See Appendix B.) Women may need natural progesterone cream, which can be obtained from a health food store, and men may need natural testosterone cream, which must be prescribed by a physician and can be compounded at a compounding pharmacy. Call Pharmacy Specialists at 1-407-260-7002 to find a physician in your area.

2. *An untreated parasitic, viral or bacterial infection*

3. *A toxic heavy metal*—such as mercury, lead or cadmium—in your system.

4. *Emotional problems* such as frustration, unforgiveness, guilt, rejection, depression or anxiety.

5. *A nutritional deficiency.* Because most candida patients cannot take a multivitamin initially in their treat-

ment, this problem may need to be addressed after other issues, such as food allergies or sensitivities, are resolved.

6. *A digestion problem.* Many candida patients have poor digestion and may need to take a digestive enzyme or a hydrochloric acid supplement. However, just as with many other supplements, this should be introduced after the initial problems are resolved.

7. *Acidosis.* Acidosis is a condition in which body tissues become overly acidic, as indicated by a urine pH test. Acidosis in the body promotes the growth of candida. For these patients, I recommend Vaxa's Buffer pH, one tablet three times a day.

8. *Excessive amounts of stress*

A BIBLE CURE HEALTH TIP

The Bible says that "a cheerful heart is good medicine, but a broken spirit saps a person's strength" (Prov.

17:22). It is a scientific fact that laughing is good for you; it releases endorphins and reduces stress levels. I recommend ten belly laughs a day in order to stimulate the immune system.

Why not go out and purchase a joke book or watch a funny movie? Learn to laugh a little more. Before you know it, everything will stop seeming so serious.

How Long Should I Stay on the Diet?

The candida diet is foundational to any good candida program. This strict diet is required for a sufficient period of time to reduce yeast overgrowth. Withholding foods on which it thrives will weaken it and allow the good bacteria to regain their important balance. The period of time varies from individual to individual due to the strength of their immune system and the severity of the disease that is being manifested.

If you have chronic fatigue or fibromyalgia, you may need to follow the candida diet for six months to a year. If you are experiencing an autoimmune disorder, you may need to be on the program for one or two years. If you are experiencing less serious symptoms of PMS, fatigue, cloudy thinking, and muscle and joint aches and pains, you may only need to be on the program three to six months.

Everyone is different, and there are a number of factors involved in determining the length of time you should stay on the candida diet. These factors include:

- The severity of the yeast overgrowth
- The strength of your immune system
- The degree of your food sensitivities
- The severity of the disease

This program involves three phases. Phase 1 is the first twenty-one days and is used to detoxify the body, break any food addictions and begin to eliminate food sensitivities. Phase 2 is an excellent program to bring candida under control, eliminate food allergies and enable you to lose weight. Phase 3 is the stabilization stage where your symptoms of candida have resolved or you have achieved your goal weight and your food sensitivities are under control. In phase 3 you can eat almost anything with the exception of foods high in sugar, highly processed foods and any other foods to which you are still sensitive or allergic.

> *Your salvation will come like the dawn. Yes, your healing will come quickly.*
> —Isaiah 58:5

Phase 1—the first three weeks

You will eat no sugar of any kind, including fruits. Also, avoid completely wheat, corn, dairy (except for a small amount of organic butter), artificial flavorings, sweeteners, food additives, yeast, vinegar, soy sauce, pickled foods, smoked or cured meats, potatoes, mushrooms, deep-fried foods, and gluten grains (such as wheat products).

Phase 2

You can add low-glycemic fruits back to your diet, such as Granny Smith apples, berries (blueberries, blackberries, raspberries, strawberries), grapefruit and kiwi. You can add all veggies except white potatoes and corn. You may be able to add oats back to your diet. See pages 9–12 for foods to avoid.

Phase 3

Add everything back to your diet except foods high in sugar and highly processed foods, as well as any foods to which you are still sensitive.

I recommend that everyone who starts the candida diet remain under the care of a good nutritional doctor who can monitor your progress. Many conventional medical doctors do not recognize candida or candida-related illnesses.

Enjoying Delicious Help

In the following chapters of this book you will find many delicious recipes that will assist you in following the candida diet. Instead of indulging in that chocolate chip cookie or piece of lemon meringue pie, you can enjoy healthy, nutritious

> *Praise the LORD, I tell myself…He forgives all my sins and heals all my diseases.*
> —PSALM 103:2–3

foods—and desserts, too—that are not only delicious, but will help restore your body to the divine health that God has for you!

A BIBLE CURE PRAYER
FOR YOU

Dear Lord, I realize that You have created my body and that You know what is best for it. I ask You for the self-control I need to maintain the nutritional guidelines I know are healthy for me and that will restore my body to a normal balance and level of functioning. Holy Spirit, help me control what I eat. Help reduce my cravings for sugar, for desserts that I should not have, and increase my desire for the foods that I should eat. Give me discipline to do the things You ask me to do so that I can walk in health all the days of my life. In Jesus' name, amen.

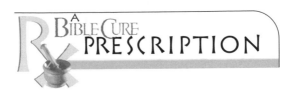

A BIBLE CURE PRESCRIPTION

Would you like to know how much of your health problem is yeast related? If so, then take the candida quiz below and add up your points to see how you stack up.[1]

1. Have you taken tetracycline or other antibiotics for acne for one month or longer? (25 points) _____
2. Have you ever taken other broad-spectrum antibiotics for respiratory, urinary or other infections for two months or longer, or in short courses four or more times in one year? (20 points) _____
3. Have you ever taken a broad-spectrum antibiotic (even a single course)? (6 points) _____
4. Have you ever been bothered by persistent prostatitis, vaginitis or other problems affecting your reproductive organs? (25 points) _____
5. Have you been pregnant one time? (3 points) _____
   Two or more times? (5 points) _____
6. Have you taken birth control pills?
   For six months to two years? (8 points) _____
   For more than two years? (15 points) _____

7. Have you taken prednisone or other cortisone-type drugs?
   For two weeks or less? (6 points) ____
   For more than two weeks? (15 points) ____
8. Does exposure to perfumes, insecticides, fabric shop odors or other chemicals provoke:
   Mild symptoms? (5 points) ____
   Moderate to severe symptoms? (20 points) ____
9. Are your symptoms worse on damp, muggy days or in moldy places? (20 points) ____
10. Have you had athlete's foot, ringworm, "jock-itch" or other chronic infections of the skin or nails?
    Mild to moderate? (10 points) ____
    Severe or persistent? (20 points) ____
11. Do you crave sugar? (10 points) ____
12. Do you crave breads? (10 points) ____
13. Do you crave alcoholic beverages? (10 points) ____
14. Does tobacco smoke really bother you? (10 points) ____

How to score the candida quiz

If you are a woman and scored over 180, yeast-connected problems are almost certainly present. If you are a man and scored over 140, yeast-connected problems are almost certainly present.

If you are a woman and scored 120–180,

yeast-connected health problems are probably present. If you are a man and scored 90–140, yeast-connected health problems are probably present.

If you are a woman and scored 60–119, yeast-connected health problems are possibly present. If you are a man and scored 40–89, yeast-connected health problems are possibly present.

If you are a woman and scored less than 60, or a man and scored less than 40, yeast-connected health problems are less likely present.

I also commonly perform a blood test to diagnose candida overgrowth. The blood test is called *Candida Immune Complexes and Antibodies*. If these tests are elevated, you should definitely begin the candida diet as well as take the supplements. Your physician can order this test by calling AAL Reference Laboratory Inc. at 1-800-552-2611.

Chapter 3

Yummy Breakfasts

California Omelet[1]
Phase 1, 2, 3

4 large organic eggs (or Egg Beaters)
1 medium avocado, scrubbed, peeled and diced
1 can (2.2-ounce) sliced ripe olives, drained (optional
1 large tomato, scrubbed and diced)
2 Tbsp. clarified butter (found in most health food stores;
  if you are unable to find, use organic butter)
2 large green onions, scrubbed, peeled and coarsely
  chopped

Beat eggs in a medium bowl with a rotary beater or electric mixer. Add other ingredients, except butter; mix. Place butter in a large skillet; melt, moving pan back and forth until entire surface and sides are coated. Add egg mixture; cook over medium heat until sides and bottom are golden brown. Turn half of omelet over other half; cover. Cook at low heat until egg is set and omelet is golden brown.

10 grams carbs; serves 2.

Scrambled Eggs Fiesta[2]
Phase 1, 2, 3

6 large organic whole eggs (or Egg Beaters)
½ cup chopped red bell peppers
1 Tbsp. minced jalapeno pepper (about 1)
1 fresh avocado, sliced
4 spelt tortillas
½ cup chopped onion
½ cup chopped green peppers
1 Tbsp. organic butter
1 can Bearitos Vegetarian Refried Black Beans
4 Tbsp. fresh salsa

Heat butter in a sauté pan and add peppers and onions; sauté until slightly soft. Scramble eggs in a separate bowl and add to pan; reduce heat and cook until eggs are scrambled.

Serve with avocado slices, salsa, refried black beans and spelt tortilla.

39 grams carbs; serves 4.

Frittata Primavera[3]
Phase 1, 2, 3

¾ Tbsp. extra-virgin olive oil (or organic butter)
½ cup chopped red bell peppers
½ cup thinly sliced onions
½ cup thinly sliced zucchini
½ cup chopped fresh tomato (liquid drained)
½ tsp. cracked black pepper

6 organic eggs, beaten
1 Tbsp. fresh basil chiffonade
1 Tbsp. fresh parsley, minced
Sea salt to taste

In a large skillet (nonstick is preferable), heat ½ Tbsp. olive oil on medium heat; add chopped red bell peppers and sauté for two minutes. Add sliced onions and sauté for 5 minutes or until soft. Add zucchini and chopped, drained tomatoes, and sauté for 2 minutes. Add cracked pepper and beaten eggs.

As eggs begin to set, loosen sides with a heat-resistant spatula. Continue to cook on medium heat (adjust heat as necessary), and cover to finish cooking the top. When top is cooked, loosen frittata and slide onto serving platter. Cut into serving portions as you would a pie. Sprinkle with sea salt if desired.

4 grams carbs; serves 3.

Poached Eggs[4]
Phase 1, 2, 3

2 poached organic eggs
2 slices spelt or millet toast
1 tsp. butter

Serves 1.

Blueberry Buckwheat Pancakes
Phase 2, 3

1 cup buckwheat pancake mix
¾ cup unsweetened soy milk
1 Tbsp. extra-virgin olive oil
1–2 cups blueberries

Heat skillet over medium-low heat.

Combine all ingredients except blueberries and stir with a wire whisk until large lumps disappear. Let stand 1–2 minutes to thicken.

Pour slightly less than ¼ cup for each pancake onto skillet, lightly greased with organic butter or extra-virgin olive oil. Sprinkle blueberries as desired on top of pancakes while cooking. Turn when pancakes bubble and bottoms are golden brown. Use sugar-free syrup made with Stevia, glycerin or sucralose.

23 grams carbs; makes 12–14 pancakes.

Millet or Rice Cereal
Phase 1, 2, 3

Use unsweetened soy, rice or almond milk with millet or rice cereal with no added sugars. You may add berries to your cereal. (This is not phase 1 if you add berries.)

Millet cereal, 77 grams carbs; rice cereal, 29 grams carbs; serves 1.

Old-Fashioned Oatmeal
Phase 2, 3

Cook your old-fashioned oatmeal in water or unsweetened soy, rice or almond milk and a small amount of organic butter. Sweeten with Stevia or Splenda. Serve with spelt or millet toast.

Serves 1.

Brown Rice Grits[5]
Phase 1, 2, 3

¼ cup dry Arrowhead Mills Rice & Shine
¾ cup water
2 tsp. organic butter, if desired
¼ cup unsweetened soy milk
1 tsp. chopped pecans
¼ tsp. cinnamon
1/16 tsp. Stevia (if extra sweetness is desired)

Add cereal to water and bring to boil, stirring constantly. Reduce heat, cover and simmer for about 2 minutes, until desired consistency is reached. Place in serving bowls and add rest of ingredients as desired to enhance grits.

CAUTION: High in carbohydrates.

6 grams carbs; serves 2.

French Toast[6]
Phase 1, 2, 3

3 whole organic eggs
¼ cup unsweetened soy milk
8 slices millet bread
½ tsp. ground nutmeg
½ tsp. ground cinnamon
1 Tbsp. organic butter

In a pie plate, whip eggs until smooth. Add soy milk, nutmeg and cinnamon. Heat butter in a sauté pan over medium heat. Briefly soak slices of bread in egg mixture and cook on both sides until golden brown. Hold on heated platter until ready to serve. Add more butter to pan as necessary. Use sugar-free syrup made with Stevia, glycerin or sucralose.

32 grams carbs; serves 4.

Chapter 4

Simple Salads

Chicken Salad[1]
Phase 1, 2, 3

2 cups finely chopped cooked chicken
½ cup finely chopped celery
2–4 chopped hard-boiled eggs
1 medium onion, chopped

Moisten with sugar/honey-free mayonnaise, obtainable from your health food store.

4 grams carbs; serves 4.

Grilled Shrimp Salad[2]
Phase 1, 2, 3

1½ lbs. medium to large shrimp, with shell and tail
   removed
2 Tbsp. olive oil
1 tsp. granulated garlic
1 tsp. cracked black pepper
¼ tsp. sea salt
1 Tbsp. chopped fresh parsley
1 lb. bag of mixed lettuce
1 cup cubed fresh tomatoes

Place raw cleaned shrimp in bowl and add olive oil, garlic, salt, pepper and fresh parsley. Coat shrimp thoroughly, marinate for 10–20 minutes. Heat broiler and place shrimp on sheet pan 4 inches from broiler and cook for 7 minutes or until they have turned pink. Do not overcook. Remove from oven and let cool slightly. (You can also grill shrimp on an outdoor grill).

Place mixed lettuce and tomatoes in a bowl and toss with ½ cup Sesame Ginger Dressing (page 41). Add shrimp, lightly toss and serve on a platter.

2½ grams carbs; serves 4.

Salad Nicoise[3]
Phase 1, 2, 3

½ head butter lettuce, broken apart
1 cup black olives, sliced
2 6-oz. cans white albacore tuna
1 cup fresh tomato, chopped
1½ cups celery, chopped
½ cup green onions, chopped
2 Tbsp. sunflower seeds
1 16-oz. can great northern beans, rinsed
2 Tbsp. chopped parsley
3 oz. Garlic Herb Dressing (page 38)
2 Tbsp. pine nuts
1 tsp. Herbs de Provence
Sea salt and cracked black pepper to taste

Combine all ingredients nicely on platter. Dress

with Garlic Herb Dressing and serve.
    17 grams carbs; serves 6.

Field Greens Salad[4]
Phase 1, 2, 3

4 oz. mixed field greens
1 fresh avocado
1 carrot, shredded
1 tomato, chopped
1 Tbsp. sunflower seeds
½ cup sunflower sprouts

Mix all ingredients in a salad bowl and toss with your choice of Lemon Grape Seed Oil Dressing (page 38) or Garlic Herb Dressing (page 38).
    11 grams carbs; serves 4.

Summer Green Salad[5]
Phase 1, 2, 3

2 medium fresh tomatoes
4 oz. fresh green beans
1 head endive, quartered and sliced
¾ cup radicchio, shredded
1 Tbsp. raw sunflower seeds
1 Tbsp. olive oil
Sea salt and cracked black pepper to taste
1 Tbsp. fresh herb mix, finely chopped

Chop fresh tomatoes. Steam green beans, and cut into 1-inch pieces. Place in salad serving bowl. Add endive, radicchio, sunflower seeds, olive oil, salt and pepper. Add finely minced fresh parsley, fresh chive, fresh mint or any mixture of your favorite fresh herbs. Toss and serve.

6 grams carbs; serves 4.

Incredible Summer Slaw[6]
Phase 2, 3

2 cups radicchio, shredded
1½ cups endive, sliced
2 cups fresh tomato, chopped
1 lb. fresh cream peas
1 small yellow banana chili pepper
¼ cup fresh cilantro, chopped
½ cup black olives, sliced
⅛ tsp. sea salt
½ tsp. cracked black pepper
2 fresh garlic cloves, minced
¼ tsp. oregano
3 Tbsp. grape seed oil
3 Tbsp. olive oil
2 Tbsp. fresh lemon juice
1 Tbsp. apple cider vinegar

Mix all ingredients in a large bowl. Toss and serve.
13 grams carbs; serves 8.

Garlic Herb Dressing[7]
Phase 2, 3

1 cup extra-virgin olive oil
¼ cup Bragg's Apple Cider Vinegar
4 Tbsp. garlic, minced
1 Tbsp. shallots, minced
3 fresh basil leaves, minced
2 tsp. fresh oregano, minced
½ tsp. thyme, minced
½ tsp. fresh parsley, minced
½ tsp. fresh tarragon, minced
½ tsp. fresh mint leaves, minced
Sea salt and cracked black pepper to taste

Mix all ingredients together in pourable container and use as a salad dressing or marinade for poultry or fish. If you prefer a creamier texture, mix ingredients in a blender or small food processor. Keep refrigerated.

This is a versatile dressing. You may substitute dried herbs for fresh, use your own choice of herbs or use lemon instead of apple cider vinegar. Add more herbs for a more intense flavor.

1 gram carbs; makes 1¾ cups.

Lemon Grape Seed Oil Dressing[8]
Phase 2, 3

½ cup grape seed oil
1 cup extra-virgin olive oil
½ cup fresh lemon juice

1 tsp. fresh lemon peel
2 tsp. garlic, chopped
2 Tbsp. shallot, chopped
¼ tsp. white pepper
½ tsp. sea salt

Place all ingredients in a pourable glass container. Shake well and dress with your favorite salad.

1 gram carbs; makes 2½ cups.

Creamy Herb Dressing[9]
Phase 2, 3

½ cup pure, cold-pressed safflower oil (from health food store)
1 large tomato, scrubbed and quartered
¼ cup fresh lemon juice
2 large cloves garlic, peeled and crushed
½ tsp. sea salt (optional)
1 Tbsp. each chopped fresh thyme and tarragon
½ tsp. ground paprika
2 Tbsp. 100 percent pure vegetable glycerine
2 Tbsp. sesame seeds

Place all ingredients in a blender, food processor or wide-mouthed jar; mix well. Refrigerate before serving.

18 grams carbs; makes approximately 1 cup.

Savory Spanish Dressing[10]
Phase 1, 2, 3

1 medium avocado, scrubbed, peeled, pitted and quartered
1 large fresh tomato, scrubbed and quartered
2 large green onions, scrubbed, peeled and cut in half
½ tsp. garlic powder
2 Tbsp. fresh lemon juice
Cayenne pepper to taste

Mix all ingredients in a food processor until creamy; pour over salad.

6 grams carbs; serves 4.

Delicious Homemade Mayonnaise[11]
Phase 2, 3

6 large, pasteurized egg yolks
2 cups pure cold-pressed safflower oil (from health food store)
¼ cup fresh lemon juice
¼ cup water (purified, preferably)
1 tsp. sea salt (optional)
1 tsp. dry mustard

Beat yolks for 2 minutes in a food processor or with an electric mixer. Pour 1 cup of the oil into a measuring cup. Very slowly drizzle a thin stream of oil from the cup into the yolks while beating at high speed until all has been used; mixture should become thick. Drizzle in remaining cup, still beating at high speed. Add lemon juice, water, salt and mustard; mix. Mayonnaise is ready! Spoon mixture into a wide-mouthed quart jar with a tight-fitting lid. Refrigerate until ready to use.

Makes approximately 3 cups.

Sesame Ginger Dressing
Phase 1, 2, 3

¼ cup cold-pressed sesame oil
¼ cup toasted sesame seeds
1½ cups olive oil
⅓ cup Bragg's Liquid Aminos
⅛ cup fresh ginger
⅛ cup fresh garlic, minced
½ Tbsp. red pepper, crushed

Mix all ingredients together and place in salad dressing cruet. Store leftover dressing in refrigerator.

1 gram carbs; makes 2½ cups.

Chapter 5

Enticing Entrées

Chicken Cutlets Italiano[1]
Phase 1, 2, 3

¼ cup extra-virgin olive oil
2 organic eggs
⅓ cup brown rice flour
4 chicken cutlets (breast halves, skinned and boned)
1 cup scrubbed zucchini, sliced in ⅛-inch rounds
1 tsp. garlic powder, more or less, to taste
1 Tbsp. chopped fresh oregano
1 8-oz. can unsweetened tomato sauce (without citric acid)

Heat oil in a large nonstick skillet. Beat eggs in a small bowl. Spoon flour into a pie dish. Dip chicken breasts first into egg, next into flour and then place in skillet; add zucchini. Sprinkle half of the seasonings over top; brown over medium-high heat. Turn; reduce heat. Spoon tomato sauce over cutlets and zucchini. Sprinkle remaining half of the seasonings over sauce. Simmer, covered, 10–15 minutes, or until fork-tender.

16 grams carbs; serves 4.

Greek-Style Breast of Chicken[2]
Phase 1, 2, 3

½ cup extra-virgin olive oil
Juice of 1 medium lemon, scrubbed before slicing
Chopped fresh oregano to taste
Garlic powder to taste
2–4 chicken breast halves, skinned, with bones

Place a small bowl and foil-lined broiling pan next to each other. Place oil, lemon juice and seasonings in bowl; mix. Dip both sides of chicken into the lemon-olive oil mixture and then place in broiling pan, reserving leftover sauce for basting. Broil one side until browned (about 5 minutes), basting often. Turn; broil other side, basting frequently until chicken is fork-tender.

2–3 grams carbs; serves 2–4.

Cajun Chicken Breast[3]
Phase 1, 2, 3

4 4-oz. boneless, skinless chicken breasts
1 Tbsp. olive oil
2 Tbsp. Cajun spice mix

Coat chicken breasts with olive oil and spice mix. Place in oven and broil for 20 minutes, turning after 10 minutes. Instead of broiling, you can also grill these chicken breasts using your favorite method.

½ grams carbs; serves 4.

Garlic Chicken and Pasta[4]
Phase 1, 2, 3

2–3 Tbsp. extra-virgin olive oil (enough for sautéing)
1 cup chicken broth
1–2 cloves garlic, minced (to taste)
1–2 Tbsp. minced onion or shallot (to taste)
Salt and pepper (to taste)
½ lemon
2 skinless chicken breasts, cut up
½ lb. cooked spelt pasta

Melt butter and olive oil in pan and sauté onion/shallot and garlic over low to medium heat until well caramelized. Add chicken and brown on all sides. Add chicken broth, salt and pepper. Lower heat and simmer until liquid is reduced by half. Squeeze ½ lemon over chicken and toss in cooked spelt pasta.

Note: For variation, add other vegetables such as squash, zucchini, broccoli, tomatoes, etc.

42 grams carbs; serves 4.

Turkey and Wild Rice Casserole[5]
Phase 1, 2, 3

1 cup raw wild rice
¼ cup extra-virgin olive oil
1 medium yellow onion, scrubbed, peeled and chopped
1 medium green bell pepper, scrubbed and diced
2 stalks celery, scrubbed and thinly sliced

¾ pound fresh natural turkey breast, cubed
8 ounces canned water chestnuts, drained and sliced
1 17½-oz. can unsweetened chicken broth
1 Tbsp. potato or brown rice flour
1 tsp. garlic powder
1 tsp. chopped fresh sage

Preheat oven to 350°. Rinse wild rice twice in colander under cold running water. Heat oil in an 8-inch nonstick skillet. Add onion, pepper, celery and turkey; sauté until browned. Add water chestnuts, rice and broth; mix. Add flour and seasonings; mix until well blended. Pour mixture into a 3-quart casserole dish. Cover; bake 45 minutes.

31 grams carbs; serves 6.

Shrimp and Chicken Jambalaya[6]
Phase 1, 2, 3

2 Tbsp. extra-virgin olive oil
4 cloves garlic, chopped
⅓ cup green onion, chopped
⅓ cup red onion, diced
⅓ cup each of yellow, red and green bell pepper, diced
¼ cup celery, diced
¼ cup fresh parsley
¼ tsp. thyme
2 cups short-grain brown rice
4¾ cups chicken stock
1¾ Tbsp. Cajun spice (read label)
3 Tbsp. butter

1¼ lb. chicken breast, cubed
1¼ lb. shrimp, peeled and deveined
Sea salt and pepper to taste

Sauté chicken and shrimp in butter and set aside in a bowl. Add salt and pepper to taste. In same pan, heat olive oil; add garlic and vegetables and sauté until translucent. Add rice and sauté for 5 minutes.

Add chicken stock and spice; cook until rice is tender. Add chicken and shrimp and toss, adding water if necessary. Serve in large bowls.

40 grams carbs; serves 6.

Orange Roughy With Special Butter Sauce and Almonds[7]
Phase 1, 2, 3

½ cup clarified or organic butter
1 tsp. each chopped fresh basil and oregano
Garlic powder to taste
4 orange roughy fillets (6–8 ounces each)
½ cup sliced or ground fresh almonds
1 medium lemon, scrubbed and cut into wedges, for garnish
Fresh parsley sprigs for garnish

Preheat oven to 350 degrees. Melt butter in a small skillet; add seasonings, mix and immediately remove from heat. Dip both sides of fish into butter sauce; place in a baking dish and pour any remaining sauce over tops of fillets. Sprinkle almonds over top. Bake 20 minutes. Test for doneness with a fork. Garnish with lemon and parsley.

7 grams carbs; serves 4.

Florentine-Stuffed Sole[8]
Phase 1, 2, 3

1 10-oz. package frozen spinach, chopped
½ cup clarified or organic butter or extra-virgin olive oil
1 tsp. garlic powder
1 tsp. each chopped fresh basil and oregano
½ tsp. ground nutmeg
4 sole fillets (6–8 ounces each)
½ cup sliced or ground fresh raw almonds
1 medium lemon, scrubbed and sliced, for garnish
Fresh parsley sprigs, for garnish

Preheat oven to 350 degrees. Thaw spinach in a microwave or colander; drain and squeeze out any liquid. Heat butter or oil in a large nonstick skillet; add spinach and seasonings. Mix well and remove from heat. Place spinach on the center of each fillet, reserving butter sauce in skillet. Roll fillets; secure with toothpicks. Place fillets into a greased 8-inch baking dish. Mix almonds into butter sauce; sprinkle over fillet tops. Bake 20 minutes; fillets are done when they flake at the touch of a fork. Garnish with lemons and parsley.

6 grams carbs; serves 4.

Meat Marinade[9]
Phase 2, 3

1 large clove garlic
2 Tbsp. lemon juice
1 Tbsp. raw unpasteurized apple cider vinegar
1½ tsp. steak spice
½ tsp. celery salt
2 Tbsp. extra-virgin olive oil
½ tsp. salt

Mix all ingredients together and coat meat before cooking. This can be used to marinate chicken breasts or on beef in a Crock-Pot. This recipe can easily be doubled.

2½ grams carbs.

Special Spaghetti and Sauce[10]
Phase 1, 2, 3

1 15-ounce can unsweetened tomato sauce (without citric acid)
1 6-ounce can tomato paste (without citric acid)
2 Tbsp. coarsely chopped fresh parsley
2 Tbsp. extra-virgin olive oil
1 Tbsp. each coarsely chopped fresh basil and oregano
1 7-oz. package cooked and drained soba, spelt or rice noodles

Place sauce ingredients in a large kettle; heat. Bring to a boil; cover and simmer 1 hour. Serve over noodles.

51 grams carbs; serves 4.

Quick Marinara Sauce[11]
Phase 1, 2, 3

2 tsp. extra-virgin olive oil
1 28-oz. can crushed tomatoes (without citric acid)
6 cloves garlic, sliced
4 fresh basil leaves
1 tsp. cracked black pepper
Sea salt to taste

Place olive oil in a saucepan and heat slightly. Add sliced garlic and sauté. Do not brown. Remove pan from heat and pour in crushed tomatoes. Place over heat again and simmer for 5 minutes. Add chopped basil leaves. Add pepper and salt to taste.

16 grams carbs; makes 3½ cups.

Hamburgers[12]
Phase 1, 2, 3

1¼ lb. lean free-range ground sirloin
1 tsp. cracked black pepper
1 tsp. Wesbrae Un-Ketchup
4 millet hamburger buns, cut in half, and grilled, broiled or toasted

Mix ingredients except buns together and divide into four 5-oz. patties. Heat broiler. Broil burgers, 4 inches from broiler, until desired doneness is reached. Approximate times: 6 minutes, rare; 8 minutes, medium rare; 10 minutes, well done. Turn burgers halfway through the cooking process.

Place burgers on buns and top with choice of sliced tomato, onion, ketchup (page 74), lettuce, pico de gallo (page 75), guacamole, pepper rings, green grilled onions or salsa. (Phase 2, add Vegenaise.)

Burgers may also be grilled or pan-fried.

40 grams carbs; serves 4.

Texas Beef and Roasted Chili[13]
Phase 1, 2, 3

2 Tbsp. extra-virgin olive oil
3 large onions, chopped
2 lb. extra-lean free range ground beef
4 Tbsp. chili powder
3 Tbsp. cumin powder
1 Tbsp. granulated garlic
1 Tbsp. cayenne pepper
1 Tbsp. cracked black pepper
1 28-oz. can crushed tomatoes (without citric acid)
3 lb. green chili peppers, roasted

In a large Crock-Pot, heat olive oil and sauté onions until translucent. Add ground beef and all spices. Cook until beef is browned. Add tomatoes and simmer for 1 hour.

In the meantime, roast chili peppers. Chop peppers, then stir into beef mixture. Heat and serve.

34 grams carbs; serves 10.

Shepherd's Pie[14]
Phase 1, 2, 3

2½ lb. lean free-range ground beef
1 Tbsp. extra-virgin olive oil
4 garlic cloves, chopped
1 cup onions, chopped
1 cup red bell pepper, chopped
1 tsp. cracked black pepper
½ tsp. garlic powder
¼ tsp. rosemary
¼ tsp. sage
¼ tsp. tarragon
2 cups petite green peas (frozen), heated
1 large head cauliflower, trimmed into florets
Pinch sea salt
¼ tsp. white pepper

In a sauté pan, brown ground beef; drain and set aside.

In the same pan, add olive oil, garlic, onions and peppers; sauté until soft. Add spices and ground beef; let simmer on low heat for about 10 minutes, then remove from heat.

Steam trimmed cauliflower until tender; drain well and pat dry. Place cauliflower in a food processor and puree until it reaches the consistency of mashed potatoes.

Season with sea salt and white pepper.

10 grams carbs; serves 8.

Braised Beef[15]
Phase 1, 2, 3

2½ lb. boneless free-range chuck roast
2 cups beef broth
1½ Tbsp. garlic, minced (about 6 cloves)
2 bay leafs
1 tsp. oregano
3 medium onions, diced
2 large celery stalks, diced
2 medium red bell peppers
1 tsp. rosemary, finely chopped
1 28-oz. can whole tomatoes, chopped in food processor
1½ tsp. cracked black pepper
¼ tsp. sea salt
2 Tbsp. extra-virgin olive oil
2 Tbsp. arrowroot (thickener)

Preheat over to 425 degrees.

Heat olive oil in roasting pan, brown roast, add vegetables, and sauté lightly about 10 minutes. Add other ingredients except arrowroot. Cover and place in oven. Cook until meat is fork tender.

Remove meat and skim fat; reduce sauce by ¼ on stovetop and thicken with arrowroot. Return meat to sauce.

For variety, try lamb, veal or pork shanks with the same preparation. (This is a great recipe for the Crock-Pot.)

19 grams carbs; serves 6.

Grilled Chicken Fajitas[16]
Phase 1, 2, 3

2 lb. boneless, skinless chicken breasts and thighs
2 Tbsp. extra-virgin olive oil
1 tsp. granulated garlic
½ tsp. sea salt
1 tsp. cracked black pepper
1 tsp. cumin powder

Cut chicken into strips. Place in bowl and add all ingredients. Marinate for 30 minutes. Heat broiler, and place chicken 4 inches from broiler. Cook for 15 minutes, turning as necessary.

Serve with warmed spelt tortillas, pico de gallo (page 75), guacamole and sautéed peppers and onions.

1 gram carbs; serves 4.

Chapter 6

Virtuous Vegetables

Spanish Brown Rice[1]
Phase 1, 2, 3

1 cup water (purified, preferably)
½ cup raw brown rice
¼ tsp. sea salt (optional)
2 Tbsp. extra-virgin olive oil
1 medium yellow onion, scrubbed, peeled and chopped
1 medium green bell pepper, scrubbed and chopped
½ cup chopped fresh parsley
2 large fresh tomatoes, scrubbed, peeled, cored and
  coarsely chopped
Cayenne pepper to taste

Bring water to a boil in a 1-quart saucepan. Add rice and salt. Reduce heat, cover and simmer 40 minutes, or until all liquid is absorbed. Heat oil in a large nonstick skillet. Add rice and rest of ingredients. Sauté over medium-high heat, stirring frequently until vegetables are tender.

26 grams carbs; serves 4.

Cajun Rice[2]
Phase 1, 2, 3

2 cups short-grain brown rice
2 Tbsp. extra-virgin olive oil
2 Tbsp. garlic, chopped
¼ cup celery, chopped
⅓ cup red bell peppers
⅓ cup yellow bell peppers
½ cup green bell peppers
¼ tsp. fresh thyme
½ tsp. crushed red pepper
1¾ Tbsp. Cajun seasoning mix
5 cups chicken broth
¼ cup parsley, chopped

Heat olive oil in a saucepan and add garlic, celery and peppers. Sauté until slightly cooked and soft. Add rice and thyme and sauté until rice is shiny, about 4 minutes. Add crushed red pepper and Cajun seasoning mix and stir. Add chicken broth and bring to a boil. Reduce heat and simmer covered for 45 minutes or until rice is cooked. Remove from heat and stir in parsley.

Note: Serve with a main meal or add to a soup or stew.

35 grams carbs; serves 10.

Wild Rice and Almonds[3]
Phase 1, 2, 3

1 cup raw wild rice
3 cups water (purified, preferably)
1 tsp. sea salt (optional)
2 Tbsp. extra-virgin olive oil
1 large clove garlic, scrubbed, peeled and minced
2 stalks celery, without leaves, scrubbed and coarsely
  chopped
1 medium yellow onion, scrubbed, peeled and coarsely
  chopped
½ cup chopped fresh parsley
½ cup slivered or ground fresh almonds

Boil wild rice with 2 cups water for 1 minute; drain. Repeat process. Then place rice, 3 cups water and salt in a 3-quart saucepan. Cover and simmer 35 minutes or until kernels puff open; drain. Pour oil into a large skillet, sauté garlic, celery, onion and parsley until tender. Add almonds and cooked rice; mix well. Simmer, covered, 15 minutes, or place rice mixture into a greased mold and bake in a preheated 350-degree oven for 20–30 minutes. Serve hot with entrée.

25 grams carbs; serves 4.

Broccoli Italian Style[4]
Phase 1, 2, 3

1 head broccoli
2 Tbsp. extra-virgin olive oil

¼ tsp. granulated garlic
⅛ tsp. sea salt
¼ tsp. cracked black pepper
¼ tsp. sesame seeds

Separate broccoli florets and cut stems to about 1½ inches or more. Steam until cooked to desired tenderness. Remove from steamer and arrange on serving platter. While still hot, drizzle olive oil over florets, then sprinkle garlic, salt, black pepper and sesame seeds over florets. Serve at room temperature.

8 grams carbs; serves 4.

Green Beans Palermo[5]
Phase 1, 2, 3

1 lb. fresh green beans
1½ tsp. extra virgin olive oil
2 garlic cloves, chopped
Sea salt and cracked black pepper to taste

Cut ends off green beans and wash thoroughly. Steam beans until desired tenderness is reached, approximately 10 minutes. Heat olive oil in sauté pan and cook garlic. Do not brown. Add green beans and toss in pan until coated. Remove from heat and place on serving dish. Add salt and pepper to taste. This dish can be served hot, cold or at room temperature.

4 grams carbs; serves 8.

Hacienda Pinto Beans[6]
Phase 1, 2, 3

2 cups dry beans* (or 2 15-oz. cans)
6 cups water (reduce 3 cups if using canned beans)
2 cups onion, chopped
4 cloves fresh garlic, chopped
2 cups fresh tomatoes, chopped
½ cup fresh cilantro, chopped
2 jalapenos, chopped
½ tsp. crushed red pepper
1 Tbsp. cumin
1 Tbsp. oregano

* Soak beans according to package directions.
In a stockpot, heat olive oil. Add onion and garlic, and sauté lightly. Add water, beans and rest of ingredients. Simmer for 2 hours. (If using canned beans, simmer for about 1 hour.)
34 grams carbs; serves 10.

Braised Cabbage and Peas[7]
Phase 1, 2, 3

1 head green cabbage (about 6 cups, sliced)
1–2 Tbsp. extra-virgin olive oil
2 Tbsp. chopped garlic
1 cup chicken broth
½ cup chopped parsley
1 cup frozen green peas
½ tsp. black pepper

Heat extra-virgin olive oil in sauté pan and add chopped garlic. Sauté garlic slightly and add cabbage. Cover and steam for 5 minutes. Add chicken broth. Reduce heat to simmer and braise for about 10 minutes. Stir in parsley and frozen peas; cover and cook for an additional 5 minutes or until the cabbage is tender. Season with pepper.

8½ grams carbs; serves 6.

Asparagus Sauté[8]
Phase 1, 2, 3

1 lb. fresh, thin asparagus, scrubbed and cut on the
  diagonal into 2-inch pieces
Water (purified, preferably)
2 Tbsp. extra-virgin olive oil
Grated, scrubbed fresh ginger root to taste
2 large cloves garlic, scrubbed, peeled and minced
½ tsp. sea salt (optional)
2 Tbsp. sesame seeds

Place asparagus in a large pot; cover with water. Bring to a boil, reduce heat, and cook 5 minutes. Heat oil in a large skillet. Add ginger, garlic, salt, sesame seeds and asparagus. Sauté, stirring and turning frequently, until tender.

3 grams carbs; serves 4.

Savory Lima Beans[9]
Phase 1, 2, 3

1 lb. dried lima beans, washed thoroughly, soaked
   overnight and drained
Water (purified, preferably)
2 Tbsp. extra-virgin olive oil
1 medium yellow onion, scrubbed, peeled and coarsely
   chopped
1 large clove garlic, scrubbed, peeled and minced
2 Tbsp. garbanzo flour
Cayenne pepper to taste
1 tsp. sea salt (optional)
1 8-oz. can unsweetened tomato sauce (without citric acid)
1 6-oz. can tomato paste (without citric acid)
1 Tbsp. 100 percent pure vegetable glycerine

Preheat oven to 350 degrees. Place beans in a large
kettle; cover with water. Bring to a boil; lower heat and
simmer 2 minutes; drain. Repeat process twice more.
Add water to cover beans; simmer covered, 30 minutes. Sauté onion and garlic in oil until tender. Place
garlic, onion, beans with liquid and rest of ingredients
in an 8-inch casserole dish; mix. Bake 45 minutes or
until tender.

23½ grams carbs; serves 6.

Chapter 7

Delicious Desserts

Tapioca Pudding[1]
Phrase 2, 3

3 Tbsp. Minute Tapioca (gluten-free)
⅛ tsp. Stevia
½ tsp. salt
2 cups unsweetened soy, almond or rice milk
1 organic egg, divided
1 tsp. vanilla

Beat egg white until light and fluffy. In a saucepan, over medium heat, combine milk, Stevia and vanilla. Heat until hot, then stir some of the soy milk into the egg yolk. Return to saucepan and add tapioca. Cook about 10 minutes, stirring constantly so it won't scorch. When thickened, fold in the egg white. Pour into four serving bowls.

8 grams carbs; serves 4.

Pumpkin and Pecan Loaf[2]
Phase 2, 3

2 large organic eggs, beaten
⅓ cup clarified or organic butter

¼ cup 100 percent pure vegetable glycerine
2 cups canned unsweetened pumpkin
1¼ cups brown rice flour
½ tsp. sea salt (optional)
2 tsp. baking powder
½ tsp. ground cloves
½ tsp. each ground cinnamon, ginger and nutmeg
½ cup chopped or ground fresh pecans

Preheat oven to 350 degrees. Mix all ingredients except nuts in a large bowl until well blended. Mix in pecans. Pour batter into a 5- x 9-inch loaf pan well oiled with extra-virgin olive oil and lightly floured. Bake 50–60 minutes. Test for doneness with a toothpick. Cool before slicing.

23 grams carbs; makes 12 slices.

Mixed Berry Compote[3]
Phase 2, 3

1 cup unsweetened blueberries, frozen
1 cup unsweetened strawberries, frozen
1 cup unsweetened blackberries, frozen
1 cup water
1⁄16 tsp. pure Stevia powder
2 tsp. arrowroot powder

Place berries and ¾ cup water in a small saucepan; cook about 15 minutes. Add Stevia, and taste for sweetness. Add more for desired sweetness, 1⁄16 tsp. at a time. Mix ¼ cup water with arrowroot powder and add to mixture; simmer until thickened. Remove from heat. Serve with pancakes or waffles.

10 grams carbs; makes 3 cups.

Dark Chocolate Almond Truffles[4]
Phase 2, 3

¾ cup almond butter
½ cup crushed almonds or pecans
3 Pure De-lite Dark Chocolate bars
¼ cup dried flaked unsweetened coconut

Line a sheet pan (or pan that can go in the freezer) with parchment paper. Freeze almond butter for 2 hours. With tip of teaspoon or melon ball tool approximately ½ teaspoon size, make small almond butter ball. Cover each ball completely with crushed almonds and place on sheet pan, leaving about 1½ inches between balls. Place back in freezer while preparing the chocolate.

Break up chocolate into 1-inch pieces. Place into a microwave-safe nonplastic container. Microwave chocolate in 40-second intervals, stirring each time, until chocolate is melted and ribbons off spoon. Do not overheat.

Take almond balls from freezer. With a teaspoon, drizzle chocolate over almond ball until the ball is completely and smoothly covered. Sprinkle with coconut, then place back in freezer until ready to serve.

5 grams carbs; makes 12 truffles, ½ oz. each.

Apple Cinnamon Bread Pudding[5]
Phase 2, 3

8 oz. green apples, sliced
1 large egg
1½ cups soy or coconut or rice milk
14 slices millet bread, cubed
¼ cup dark agave nectar
½ tsp. cinnamon
¼ tsp. allspice
¼ tsp. ginger
½ tsp. butter to coat baking pan

Mix egg, milk and spices until incorporated. Add cubed bread and soak until mixture is absorbed. Add more milk if too dry. Fold in apples. Place in buttered glass baking dish. Bake at 350 degrees for 25 minutes until top is browned.

40 grams carbs; serves 6.

Lemon and Pecan Cookies[6]
Phase 2, 3

½ cup clarified or organic butter
3 Tbsp. 100 percent pure vegetable glycerine
1 large organic egg
1½ cups + 4½ tsp. brown rice flour
½ tsp. baking soda
¼ cup fresh lemon juice
2 Tbsp. lemon flavoring
½ cup chopped or ground pecans

Preheat oven to 375 degrees. Mix butter and glycerine in a large bowl. Add egg, flour and baking soda; mix well. Fold in lemon juice, flavoring and pecans. Drop rounded teaspoonfuls of dough onto a nonstick cookie sheet. Bake 8–10 minutes. Cool 5 minutes before removing from cookie sheet.

12 grams carbs; makes 2 dozen cookies.

Nut Butter Cookies[7]
Phase 2, 3

¼ cup clarified or organic butter, melted
½ cup Delicious and Easy Nut Butter (page 79)
2 Tbsp. 100 percent pure vegetable glycerine
⅓ cup unsweetened soy milk
1 large organic egg
1 tsp. vanilla flavoring
1¼ cups sifted brown rice flour
1 tsp. baking powder
¼ tsp. sea salt (optional)
2 dozen fresh pecans or walnuts, cut into halves or ground

Preheat oven to 350 degrees. Combine butters, glycerine, milk, egg and flavoring in a large bowl. Place dry ingredients in another large bowl; mix together. Add dry mixture to milk mixture; blend well. Place teaspoonfuls of dough on a nonstick cookie sheet; flatten cookies with back of spoon; press nut halves into tops. Bake 8–10 minutes. Let cookies cool for 5 minutes before removing them from cookie sheet. Cookies will harden as they cool.

5 grams carbs; makes 4 dozen cookies.

Pumpkin Cookies[8]
Phase 2, 3

1 cup canned unsweetened pumpkin
½ cup clarified or organic butter
¼ cup 100 percent pure vegetable glycerine
1 Tbsp. orange flavoring
1½ cups brown rice flour
1 tsp. baking soda
1 tsp. ground cinnamon
¼ tsp. sea salt (optional)
½ cup chopped or ground fresh walnuts

Preheat oven to 375°. Mix pumpkin, butter, glycerine and orange flavoring in a large bowl. Add flour, baking soda and seasonings; mix. Fold in nuts. Place teaspoonfuls on a nonstick cookie sheet. Bake 8–10 minutes or until lightly browned. Let cookies stand for 5 minutes before removing them from cookie sheet. They will harden as they cool.

8 grams carbs; makes 3 dozen cookies.

Chapter 8

Scrumptious Soups, Snacks and Appetizers

Savory Black Bean Soup[1]
Phase 1, 2, 3

1 cup raw black beans, washed thoroughly, soaked
   overnight and drained
1 quart water (purified, preferably)
1 Tbsp. coarsely chopped fresh parsley
¾ tsp. ground turmeric
⅛ tsp. ground cumin
1 tsp. each chopped fresh marjoram and thyme
2 Tbsp. extra-virgin olive oil
2 large cloves garlic, scrubbed, peeled and minced
1 medium yellow onion, scrubbed, peeled and finely
   chopped
2 stalks celery, without leaves, scrubbed and finely chopped
1 6-oz. can tomato paste (without citric acid)
Sea salt to taste (optional)

   Place beans in a large kettle; cover with water.
Bring to a boil; cook 2 minutes; drain. Repeat boiling
process twice more. Then place 1 quart water, beans,
spices and herbs in kettle; bring to a boil. Simmer

67

uncovered, 30 minutes. Spoon beans and their liquid into blender; blend until creamy. Place mixture in kettle; bring to a boil; simmer, uncovered. Heat oil in a small skillet. Sauté garlic and onion until tender; add with tomato paste to beans. Mix; cook uncovered 10 minutes and serve.

29 grams carbs; serves 6.

Lentil Soup and Meatballs[2]
Phase 1, 2, 3

3 Tbsp. olive oil
3 celery stalks, chopped
1 large onion, chopped
3 cloves garlic, chopped
8 cups water
2 cups lentils (washed and rinsed thoroughly)
1 tsp. thyme
1 tsp. sea salt
1 tsp. cracked black pepper
1 cup baby spinach

Heat olive oil in stockpot. Add celery, onion and garlic; sauté until tender. Add water, lentils and spices. Simmer until the lentils are tender—approximately 1 hour. Add spinach and meatballs; simmer for 15 minutes.

Meatballs:
½ lb. ground sirloin, pork or veal
1 tsp. cracked black pepper

½ tsp. sea salt
¼ tsp. crushed red pepper

Mix all ingredients thoroughly in a bowl. Form into small ½-inch meatballs and drop into simmer soup.

23 grams carbs; serves 10.

Minestrone[3]
Phase 1, 2, 3

2 Tbsp. olive oil
4 cloves garlic, chopped
1 medium onion, chopped
2 celery stalks with leaves, chopped
2 cups green cabbage
1 28-oz. can whole tomatoes, chopped in food processor
4 cups water (more or less for desired heartiness of soup)
2 cups fresh baby spinach
¼ cup fresh basil, chopped
¼ cup fresh parsley, chopped
1 tsp. rosemary
¼ tsp. oregano
1 can white beans, rinsed
Sea salt and cracked black pepper to taste

Heat olive oil in stockpot. Add garlic, onion, celery and cabbage; sauté until vegetables are tender. Add tomatoes, water and spices; simmer for 30–45 minutes. Add spinach and white beans. Stir and simmer for 5 minutes until spinach is wilted and soup is thoroughly heated.

16 grams carbohydrates per serving; serves 12.

Chicken and Rice Soup[4]
Phase 1, 2, 3

1 chicken, skinned and cut up
2 quarts water or broth
4 cloves garlic, sliced (optional, to taste)
2 cups each celery, carrots, onions, peas (sliced)
½ cup cooked brown rice
½ cup parsley, chopped
Herbs and seasoning to taste

Simmer chicken in water or stock for 40 minutes. Add vegetables and rice; simmer for 20 additional minutes. Serve broth and vegetables with chicken meat. Top with scissor-snipped fresh parsley. Add herbs according to taste.

Variation: ¼ cup raw rice may be added to water and simmered with chicken.

12 grams carbs; serves 10.

Gazpacho Soup[5]
Phase 1, 2, 3

3 cups tomato juice (read labels)
6 cups V-8 juice (low sodium, read label)
1 Tbsp. cracked black pepper
1 tsp. sea salt
¼ tsp. cayenne pepper
¼ cup olive oil
2 cups beef stock (can use vegetable or chicken stock)

1 Tbsp. ground cumin
1 tsp. Bragg's Amino Acid
2 tsp. chili powder
2 tsp. minced garlic
2 Tbsp. fresh cilantro, chopped (for garnish)
1 cucumber, chopped (for garnish)

Combine all ingredients in food processor and pulse until combined. Place in large bowl and chill for 2 hours. Serve in chilled bowls.

9 grams carbs; serves 12.

Guacamole[6]
Phase 1, 2, 3

16 oz. avocados or 1 pkg. Hass Avocado Halves
8-oz. pkg. Avo Green Salsa
2 Tbsp. fresh cilantro, chopped
1 small fresh tomato, chopped
½ small red onion, chopped
Sea salt

Crush avocados and mix in all ingredients or pulse in food processor. Add sea salt to taste.

5 grams carbs; makes 2½ cups.

Black Bean Dip[7]
Phase 1, 2, 3

1 15-oz. can black beans (drained and rinsed)
2 medium fresh tomatoes, chopped
½ cup cilantro, chopped

⅓ cup white onion, chopped
2 small serrano peppers, minced
1 Tbsp. lime juice

Place all ingredients in food processor and process until desired consistency is reached.

11 grams carbs; serves 6.

Hummus[8]
Phase 1, 2, 3

1 15-oz. chickpeas (garbanzo beans), drained
2 Tbsp. olive oil
1 Tbsp. sesame oil
¼ tsp. cracked black pepper
1 tsp. fresh garlic
2 Tbsp. water

Mix all ingredients in a small food processor until smooth. Serve with Belgian endive or Edward & Sons Brown Rice Crackers.

11 grams carbs; serves 8.

Garlic Bread[9]
Phase 2, 3

16 thinly sliced ¼-inch "O" spelt sourdough bread
½ tsp. extra-virgin olive oil
¼ tsp. granulated garlic
¼ tsp. cracked black pepper
¼ tsp. oregano
¼ tsp. red pepper, crushed

Place bread on sheet pan, spray with olive oil, and sprinkle each slice with spice mixture. Place about 4 inches from broiler and broil for about 3–4 minutes until browned.

22 grams carbs; serves 8.

Quinoa Tabouli[10]
Phase 1, 2, 3

1½ cup quinoa
2 medium cucumbers, skinned, seeded and chopped
½ cup fresh parsley, chopped
2 Tbsp. fresh lemon juice
1 tsp. fresh garlic, chopped
1 Tbsp. olive oil
Sea salt and pepper

Cook quinoa according to package directions. Let cool. Add cucumbers, parsley, lemon juice, garlic, olive oil, salt and pepper. Mix all ingredients thoroughly and chill.

47 grams carbs; serves 4.

Chapter 9

And That's Not All!

Ketchup[1]
Phase 1, 2, 3

1 cup Westbrae Unsweetened Un-Ketchup
$\frac{1}{16}$ tsp. pure Stevia powder

Mix to combine ingredients. Use as you would regular ketchup.

0 grams carbs; serves 4.

Almond Milk[2]
Phase 2, 3

1 cup fresh raw almonds
2 cups boiling water (purified, preferably)
1 quart cold water (purified, preferably)
1 Tbsp. pure, cold-pressed safflower oil from health food store
2 Tbsp. 100 percent pure vegetable glycerine
$\frac{1}{4}$ tsp. sea salt (optional)

Blanch almonds by pouring boiling water over nuts; soak a few minutes or until skins slide off easily; drain. Place skinless almonds, cold water, oil, glycerine and salt in a food processor or blender. Process to a very smooth liquid. If necessary, strain with cheesecloth or a fine strainer; refrigerate. Use in recipes as you would pasteurized or soy milk.

4 grams carbs; makes approximately 1 quart.

Mock Sour Cream[3]
Phase 2, 3

1 cup plain low-fat, lactose-free yogurt
1 tsp. 100 percent pure vegetable glycerine

Mix yogurt and glycerine in a small bowl. Chill at least 30 minutes before serving.

12 grams carbs; makes approximately 1 cup.

Pico de Gallo[4]
Phase 1, 2, 3

2½ cups fresh tomatoes, diced
1 cup onion, diced
½ cup cilantro, chopped
½ cup serrano peppers, minced
Pinch sea salt
Squeeze of lemon juice

Mix all ingredients in a bowl. Chill and serve as a condiment with beans and fajitas.

5 grams carbs; serves 4–6.

Béarnaise II Sauce[5]
Phase 2, 3

1½ Tbsp. Bragg's Apple Cider Vinegar
1 shallot, finely minced
½ tsp. cracked black pepper
1½ Tbsp. tarragon
2 Tbsp. lemon juice
½ cup clarified butter
3 organic egg yolks
1½ Tbsp. water
½ tsp. sea salt

In a small saucepan over medium heat, combine apple cider vinegar, shallot, pepper, tarragon, lemon juice and ½ Tbsp. water. Simmer until reduced by ⅓. Remove from heat.

In the upper section of a double boiler, off heat, whisk egg yolks and cold water until frothy. Place the pan over the barely simmer water of the bottom section and continue whisking egg yolks for 3–4 minutes until eggs are thickened. Do not let eggs get too hot or they will scramble.

When eggs are thickened, remove pan from heat and slowly whisk in warm clarified butter. Whisk in the reduced tarragon liquid until sauce is smooth and incorporated. Keep covered until ready to serve.

1 gram carbs; makes 1 cup.

Cocktail Sauce[6]
Phase 1, 2, 3

1 cup Westbrae Unsweetened Un-Ketchup
1/16 tsp. white Stevia powder
1/2 tsp. Bragg's Amino Acids
1 Tbsp. organic horseradish

Mix all ingredients together in a bowl. Garnish with fresh herbs. Use more or less horseradish to your taste.

10 grams carbs; serves 6.

Cajun Nut Mix[7]
Phase 1, 2, 3

1 cup raw hulled sunflower seeds
1 cup soy nuts
1 cup pecan halves
1 cup pumpkin seeds
1 cup almonds
1 Tbsp. Cajun seasoning mix (be sure to check the label for "illegal" additives)
Extra-virgin olive oil
Sea salt

Preheat oven to 350 degrees. Lightly spray olive oil onto a sheet pan. Place nuts and seeds on pan, and spray them lightly with olive oil. Sprinkle seasoning and salt to lightly coat mixture. Roast mixture until lightly browned, approximately 15 minutes. Turn halfway through the cooking process. Remove from oven and reseason. Let cool completely. Place in glass bowl or jar. Store in airtight container and refrigerate.

40 grams carbs; 10-plus servings.

Salt-Free Chili Powder[8]
Phase 1, 2, 3

2 Tbsp. paprika
2 tsp. oregano
1¼ tsp. ground cumin
1¼ tsp. garlic powder
¾ tsp. cayenne pepper
¾ tsp. onion powder

Combine all ingredients; mix thoroughly. Store in airtight container.

1 gram carbs per teaspoon; makes ¼ cup.

Creole Seasoning[9]
Phase 1, 2, 3

8 tsp. salt
2 Tbsp. pepper
2 Tbsp. garlic powder
8 tsp. paprika
8 tsp. cayenne pepper
4½ tsp. onion powder
1 Tbsp. thyme
2 Tbsp. grated lemon rind

In a screw-top jar, combine all ingredients. Shake thoroughly to mix. Keep in a dry place.

¾ grams carbs; makes ¾ cup.

Delicious and Easy Nut Butter[10]
Phase 1, 2, 3

½ cup fresh raw pecans, walnuts or almonds
1 tablespoon cold-pressed safflower oil (from health food
  store)

Combine nuts and oil in a food processor or blender; mix until creamy. Spread on rice cakes or rice crackers or use in recipes.

1¾ grams carbs per teaspoon

Appendix A

Passport Life Program

Ed McClure weighed over 450 pounds before he was educated about candida and placed on the candida diet. Since implementing the diet and taking the required supplements, he has now lost over 200 pounds. This success filled Ed with a passion to help others suffering from candida. Ed and his wife, Elise, have developed The Passport Life Program in which he teaches seminars on how to overcome candida. For more information on this wonderful program, please visit their Web site at www.passportlife.com.

Appendix B

Ordering Information for Supplements

Vaxa Buffer pH
1-877-622-8292
Provide #R.S. 49466

Divine Health Candida Formula
www.drcolbert.com

Divine Health Probiotic
www.drcolbert.com

Moducare
From most health food stores

NAET
To find a doctor in your area who performs NAET,
   visit their Web site at www.naet.com.

Natur-Leaf
1-888-532-7845

Nystatin
Call your physician or Pharmacy Specialists at 1-407-260-7002 to find a physician.

Probiotic Pearls
Integrative Therapeutics at 1-800-931-1709
When prompted, provide Dr. Colbert's PCP #5266

Total Leaky Gut by Nutri-West
1-800-451-5620

Three Lac
1-760-542-3000
Provide #ID 40274

ALCAT
This test must be performed by a physician.
1-800-881-2685

DSF
Nutri-West
1-800-451-5620

A Personal Note From
Don and Mary Colbert

God's Word is full of promises that confirm His love for you and His desire to give you His abundant life. His desire includes more than physical health for you; He wants to make you whole in your mind and spirit as well through a personal relationship with His Son, Jesus Christ.

If you haven't met our best friend, Jesus, we would like to take this opportunity to introduce Him to you. It is very simple.

Just bow your head and sincerely pray this prayer from your heart:

> *Lord Jesus, I want to know You as my Savior and Lord. I believe You are the Son of God and that You died for my sins. I ask You to forgive me for my sins and change my heart so that I can be Your child and live with You eternally. Thank You for Your peace. Help me to walk with You so that I can begin to know You as my best friend and my Lord. Amen.*

If you have prayed this prayer, we rejoice with you in your decision and your new relationship with Jesus. Please contact us at pray4me@strang.com so that we can send you some materials that will help you become established in your relationship with the Lord. You have just made the most important decision of your life. We look forward to hearing from you.

Notes

Chapter 2

1. Adapted from William G. Crook, *The Yeast Connection Handbook* (Jackson, TN: Professional Books, 1999), 15–19.

Chapter 3

1. Gail Burton, *The Candida Control Cookbook* (Fairfield, CT: Aslan Publishing, 1995), 59.
2. Ed and Elisa McClure, *Eat Your Way to Heal-Thy Life* (Boerne, TX: Passport Life Center), 92. Ed and Lisa are founders of Passport Life Center. Visit their Web site at www.passportlife.com. Used by permission.
3. Ibid., 93.
4. Ibid., 95.
5. Ibid., page not given.
6. Ibid.

Chapter 4

1. Crook, *The Yeast Connection Handbook*, 222.
2. McClure, *Eat Your Way to Heal-Thy Life*.
3. Ibid., 44.
4. Ibid., 35.
5. Ibid., 38.
6. Ibid., 45.
7. Ibid., page not given.
8. Ibid., 41.
9. Burton, *The Candida Control Cookbook*, 144.
10. Ibid.

11. Ibid., 145.

CHAPTER 5

1. Burton, *The Candida Control Cookbook*, 82.
2. Ibid., 85.
3. McClure, *Eat Your Way to Heal-Thy Life*.
4. Ibid.
5. Burton, *The Candida Control Cookbook*, 91.
6. McClure, *Eat Your Way to Heal-Thy Life*, 62.
7. Burton, *The Candida Control Cookbook*, 72.
8. Ibid., 69.
9. Karen Tripp, *Candida Recipe Collection*, as viewed at http://www.geocities.com/HotSprings/4966/marinade.htm.
10. Burton, *The Candida Control Cookbook*, 103.
11. McClure, *Eat Your Way to Heal-Thy Life*.
12. Ibid., 46.
13. Ibid., 47.
14. Ibid., 50.
15. Ibid., 52.
16. Ibid., 53.

CHAPTER 6

1. Burton, *The Candida Control Cookbook*, 110.
2. McClure, *Eat Your Way to Heal-Thy Life*.
3. Burton, *The Candida Control Cookbook*, 112.
4. McClure, *Eat Your Way to Heal-Thy Life*, 75.
5. Ibid., 73.
6. Ibid., 72.
7. Ibid., page not given.
8. Burton, *The Candida Control Cookbook*, 119.

9. Ibid., 125.

Chapter 7

1. Tripp, Candida Recipe Collection as viewed at http://www.geocities.com/HotSprings/4966/tapioca.htm.
2. Burton, *The Candida Control Cookbook*, 152.
3. McClure, *Eat Your Way to Heal-Thy Life*, 85.
4. Ibid., 86.
5. Ibid., 87.
6. Burton, *The Candida Control Cookbook*, 186.
7. Ibid., 187.
8. Ibid., 189.

Chapter 8

1. Burton, *The Candida Control Cookbook*, 54.
2. McClure, *Eat Your Way to Heal-Thy Life*, 32.
3. Ibid., 33.
4. *Candida Albicans Yeast-Free Cookbook*, 63.
5. McClure, *Eat Your Way to Heal-Thy Life*, 30.
6. Ibid., 16.
7. Ibid., 17.
8. Ibid.
9. Ibid., 18.
10. Ibid., 19

Chapter 9

1. McClure, *Eat Your Way to Heal-Thy Life*, 21.
2. Burton, *The Candida Control Cookbook*, 38.
3. Ibid., 40.
4. McClure, *Eat Your Way to Heal-Thy Life*, 25.
5. Ibid., 29.

6. Ibid., page not given.
7. Ibid.
8. Karen Tripp in Chyrel's Kitchen as viewed at http://www/linkline.com/personal/gingen/season/chilifre.htm.
9. Ibid., as viewed at http://www/linkline.com/personal/gingen/season/creole2.htm.
10. Burton, *The Candida Control Cookbook*, 37.

Don Colbert, M.D., was born in Tupelo, Mississippi. He attended Oral Roberts University School of Medicine in Tulsa, Oklahoma, where he received a bachelor of science degree in biology in addition to his degree in medicine. Dr. Colbert completed his internship and residency with Florida Hospital in Orlando, Florida. He is board certified in family practice and has received extensive training in nutritional medicine.

If you would like more
information about natural and
divine healing, or information about
Divine Health Nutritional Products,
you may contact
Dr. Colbert at:

<u>Dr. Don Colbert</u>
1908 Boothe Circle
Longwood, FL 32750
Telephone: 407-331-7007
(For ordering products only)
Dr. Colbert's Web site is
www.drcolbert.com

Disclaimer: Dr. Colbert and the staff of Divine Health Wellness Center are prohibited from addressing a patient's medical condition by phone, facsimile or e-mail. Please refer questions related to your medical condition to your own primary care physician.